Electronic Fetal Heart Rate Monitoring

To Gillian and Eleanor

Electronic Fetal Heart Rate Monitoring

A Practical Guide

Paul L. Wood
H. Gordon Dobbie

Department of Obstetrics and Gynaecology
University of Leicester Medical School, Leicester, UK

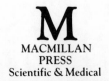

MACMILLAN
PRESS
Scientific & Medical

First published 1989

Published by
THE MACMILLAN PRESS LTD
Houndmills, Basingstoke, Hampshire RG21 2XS
and London
Companies and representatives
throughout the world

Printed in Hong Kong

British Library Cataloguing in Publication Data
Wood, Paul L.
1. Man. Foetuses. Heart rate monitoring
Electronic fetal heart rate monitoring.
I. Title II. Dobbie, H. Gordon
618.3′20754
ISBN 0–333–47117–2
ISBN 0–333–47118–0 Pbk

Contents

Contents

Foreword

'The fetal heart just stopped.' This was often the conclusion reached when intermittent auscultation of the fetal heart during labour was the only way to assess fetal well-being. It occurred apparently without warning and with often nothing to suggest a sudden accident such as abruption of the placenta or prolapse of the cord.

The ability to record the fetal heart rate continuously gave the obstetrician the opportunity to appreciate that in the majority of instances the fetal heart does not suddenly stop, but that warning signs are present in the pattern of the fetal heart rate before fetal death. Since anoxia is the basic problem, it was also anticipated that not only could intrauterine deaths be avoided, but also the birth of severely asphyxiated babies.

Whether or not the results have lived up to the expectations of the new innovation is open to question. Its use has certainly led to a greater incidence of operative deliveries, but unfortunately without a corresponding decrease in the numbers of perinatal deaths related to anoxia.

What is clear now is that the value of continuous fetal heart recording depends on three separate factors, and unless they are all satisfactory, the exercise is worse than useless. Too many errors have been made by misinterpretation of good records or by attempting to interpret bad traces.

Firstly, the machine used must be of good quality. There is no point in using a machine that, due to age or for other technical reasons, gives a poor record.

Secondly, the person in charge of the investigation must be aware of what is required and should not leave a trace to sort itself out. Twenty minutes' continuous attendance on the patient may save time in the long run by achieving a meaningful result. It must also be recognised that in the very stout patient the exercise may be difficult and unsatisfactory, and for this reason impractical.

Finally, the person interpreting the trace must understand what is of significance in a recording and what is not. It is as important to recognise normality as abnormality and to know the pitfalls in diagnosis.

It is for those who need to interpret fetal cardiotocography that this book is written. Such a practical guide is the summation of the experience of two obstetricians in daily contact with clinical situations over several years, who have had the advantage of studying the fetal outcome, following decisions made on fetal cardiotocography both antenatally and in labour.

Although the book is intended for the houseman and midwife, anyone who practises obstetrics would find the time spent browsing through it well worth while. It should help to obviate errors in the interpretation of continuous fetal cardiotocographs, which can not only bring the technique into disrepute, but also lead to mistakes in clinical management.

John MacVicar
Professor of Obstetrics and Gynaecology
University of Leicester Medical School

Preface

Electronic fetal monitoring is commonly and often routinely used in many delivery suites. The newly appointed obstetric houseman is often asked to interpret changes in FHR patterns on the basis of little prior experience. This manual aims to provide an insight into normal cardiotocography, and, while the authors accept that the interpretation of abnormal traces is far from achieving a consensus view, we aim to alert at an early stage both junior hospital doctors and midwifery staff to cardiotocographic features that merit further action. It is not intended to advocate universal cardiotocography and it is important to realise that it may form only part of the overall evaluation of the fetus, both antenatally and intrapartum. Emphasis is given to the practical problems encountered rather than to the underlying theoretical considerations, which are amply covered in other reference texts.

The cardiotocographs chosen are therefore accompanied where relevant by appropriate pH values of scalp or umbilical artery blood, Apgar scores and fetal outcome. Important points are highlighted within individual boxes and bear relevance to the accompanying text. Advice is also given as to what basic measures should be taken in the presence of an abnormal trace.

The book is intended to fill a basic gap which is often encountered in the labour ward by inexperienced staff; we hope it will not only improve fetal outcome but also prevent unnecessary intervention.

Cardiotocography as such will be of value only if the human monitor supervising the electronic monitor has a basic understanding of its interpretation.

Leicester, 1988

P.L.W.
H.G.D.

──────1──────

Purpose and Rationale of Fetal Heart Rate Monitoring

Purpose

This is to detect at an early stage inadequate fetal oxygenation, either antenatally or intrapartum, thus anticipating an abnormal outcome for the neonate and enabling the obstetrician to intervene and deliver the baby before permanent damage is done. It is hoped that in this way fetal heart rate monitoring will reduce intrapartum asphyxia and stillbirths.

Rationale

WHY DO WE MONITOR THE FETAL HEART?

Fetal heart rate monitoring is used as a clinical tool to detect fetal hypoxia, and its value in this respect depends largely on the equation:

$$\text{Cardiac output} = \text{Heart rate} \times \text{Stroke volume}$$

There is however an important difference between adult and fetus in the relationship of cardiac output, heart rate and stroke volume. In the adult an increase in cardiac output can be achieved by increasing both heart rate and stroke volume. An increase in stroke volume in the adult occurs as a result of the Frank–Starling mechanism, whereby the amount of blood pumped out by the heart depends on the amount of blood entering it; i.e. as more blood flows into the heart, the cardiac muscle contracts harder in order to pump it out, thus increasing the cardiac output. In the fetus the Frank–Starling mechanism is much less well developed and this means that as the fetus is unable to increase its stroke volume to any great extent, the fetal cardiac output is mainly dependent on heart rate.

> In the fetus, cardiac output and
> thus the oxygen supply to the
> brain are mainly heart-rate
> dependent.

FACTORS CONTROLLING FETAL HEART RATE (FHR)

The average FHR is 140 beats per minute (b.p.m.) and is greater earlier in pregnancy. For example,

average FHR at 20 weeks = 155 b.p.m.;
average FHR at 30 weeks = 144 b.p.m..

From around the twentieth week of gestation, variations occur in the FHR from beat to beat and good variability of FHR is an important sign of fetal well-being.

As outlined in Fig. 1.1, many physiological factors can affect the fetal heart rate. The cardioregulatory centre, situated in the medulla oblongata, receives impulses from different sources that help to modulate the intrinsic FHR.

Baroreceptors

These are stretch receptors that are sensitive to change in blood pressure and are situated in the arch of the aorta and in the carotid sinus. In response to a rise in blood pressure, impulses from the baroreceptors are sent to the cardioregulatory centre, resulting in an increase in vagal stimulation. This therefore slows the heart rate in an attempt to restore the blood pressure to a normal level.

Chemoreceptors

These are situated in the carotid and aortic bodies, in a similar position to that of the baroreceptors, and also in the midbrain itself. The chemoreceptors respond to changes in oxygen and carbon dioxide tensions. A fall in oxygen tension (pO_2) in blood detected by the carotid and aortic bodies would result in a sympathetic discharge from the cardioregulatory centre. This causes an increase in FHR and thus blood pressure. If the fall in pO_2 was severe, then diversion of blood from the gut, liver and kidney to the vital organs, the brain and the heart, would also result.

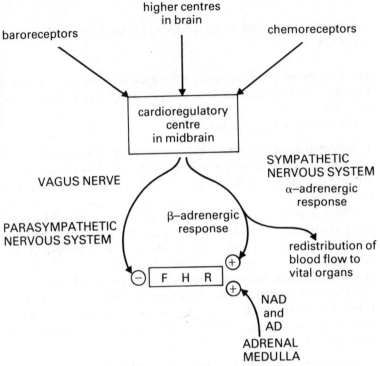

Fig. 1.1   Control of fetal heart rate

Adrenal medullary response

In response to stress the adrenal medulla releases the hormones noradrenaline (NAD) and adrenaline (AD), which results in an increase in both FHR and the force of cardiac contraction, in a manner similar to sympathetic nerve stimulation.

Higher centres in the brain

There are influences on the cardioregulatory centre from higher centres in the brain. It is this input that is thought to be responsible for the so-called fetal rest–activity cycles. During a fetal rest cycle the fetus is apparently sleeping in utero with fetal body and limb movements, electroencephalogram activity and FHR variability all decreased. A fetal rest cycle normally lasts about 20 minutes, following which there is a return to normal fetal movements and FHR variability.

    The intrinsic FHR is therefore under the complex influence of many physiological factors and is modulated by the parasympathetic and sympathetic nervous systems (as outlined in Fig. 1.1).

EFFECT OF HYPOXIA/ASPHYXIA ON THE FETUS

The fetal brain is very sensitive to oxygen deprivation and under stressful situations certain fetal compensatory mechanisms come into play.

In response to hypoxaemia:

1. Stimulation of the sympathetic nervous system and increased adrenal medullary activity result in an increased heart rate in an attempt to increase cardiac output and redistribution of blood flow to vital organs.

2. There is an increase in breakdown of liver glycogen to supply energy to the fetus. As a result of this anaerobic metabolism there is an accumulation of lactic acid to produce a metabolic acidosis. Although initially the acidosis is compensated by fetal buffering systems, especially haemoglobin, this will eventually be overcome and the acidosis will become more severe. When the pH drops below 7.0, enzyme systems, e.g. glycolysis, are inhibited, and this level of acidosis, if maintained, will therefore not be compatible with survival.

The length of time that a fetus can withstand hypoxia is related to its glycogen reserves. This means that a growth-retarded fetus with low glycogen stores will be more susceptible to intrauterine asphyxia.

Factors that can cause fetal hypoxaemia and are commonly encountered are outlined in Table 1.1. The FHR patterns found in association with these factors and their interpretation are discussed in Chapter 5.

Electronic FHR monitoring is a useful screening test. Unfortunately there is often great difficulty in the interpretation of FHR traces as they do not always accurately reflect fetal oxygenation. Overinterpretation of abnormal FHR traces is the main reason for the increased intervention rates associated with electronic FHR monitoring. It is for this reason that fetal scalp blood sampling (FBS) is employed where difficulty is found in the interpretation of an abnormal FHR pattern. There is a good correlation between fetal scalp pH taken just prior to delivery and umbilical cord pH and therefore it would seem that fetal scalp pH is a reliable indicator of fetal acidosis.

Table 1.1 Factors that commonly cause fetal hypoxaemia

---

1. Reduction in uterine blood flow:
   — uterine contractions;
   — uterine hyperstimulation, e.g. overstimulation with oxytocin or in association with abruptio placentae;
   — fall in maternal blood pressure, e.g. supine hypotension, hypovolaemic shock, epidural analgesia;
   — placental insufficiency, e.g. secondary to hypertension.
2. Reduction in umbilical blood flow, e.g. compression of umbilical cord.

A fetal blood sample can normally be obtained once the membranes are ruptured, the cervix is at least 3 cm dilated and the presenting part is in the pelvis.

The procedure is fairly standard. An amnioscope is passed transcervically and held against the fetal scalp, which is cleaned with a swab or cotton wool ball. The scalp is sprayed with ethyl chloride to produce a reactive hyperaemia and then a thin layer of silicone gel is applied which allows containment of a droplet of blood. The droplet of blood is obtained by making a small incision in the scalp and the blood is then collected by capillary action in a heparinised glass capillary tube. Pressure is then applied to the fetal scalp for a short time to ensure haemostasis.

A fetal scalp pH ≥ 7.25 is considered normal and labour could continue. Where the pH is < 7.20 delivery of the baby is indicated. Where the pH is in the range 7.20 to 7.25, this is considered pre-acidotic and the sample should be repeated within 30 minutes.

> Fetal scalp sampling is a necessary and important backup to electronic FHR monitoring to avoid unnecessary caesarean sections due to misdiagnosis of fetal distress.

2

Equipment

The fetal monitor has two basic functions: to monitor the fetal heart rate and to assess uterine activity.

The Fetal Heart

The fetal heart may be monitored externally via a Doppler ultrasound transducer applied to the maternal abdomen or directly via an electrode applied to the fetal scalp (Fig. 2.1).

EXTERNAL (INDIRECT) FHR MONITORING

This method has the advantage of being simple to use and easy to apply and does not require rupture of the membranes. An ultrasound transducer is applied to the maternal abdomen and held in place by a belt. A coupling gel is required between the transducer and the maternal skin as a continuous beam of ultrasound is transmitted via the transducer through the maternal abdomen to the fetal heart. If the fetal heart was stationary then the ultrasound waves would be reflected back at the frequency they were transmitted at. However, because the fetal heart is a moving object the frequency of the reflected waves is different. This change in frequency is called the Doppler effect and these frequency changes are what the FHR monitor detects as cardiac movement.

Unfortunately, one drawback with this system has been the level of interference brought about by movements in addition to those of the heart wall and valves (e.g. fetal chest wall, body movements, blood flow through various fetal organs) which obscure the FHR, often giving a false impression of the level of variability.

Another disadvantage of external ultrasound monitoring is that during labour it tends to be unreliable because of maternal and fetal movements, requiring frequent adjustment to the position of the transducer on the maternal abdomen. In the latest generation

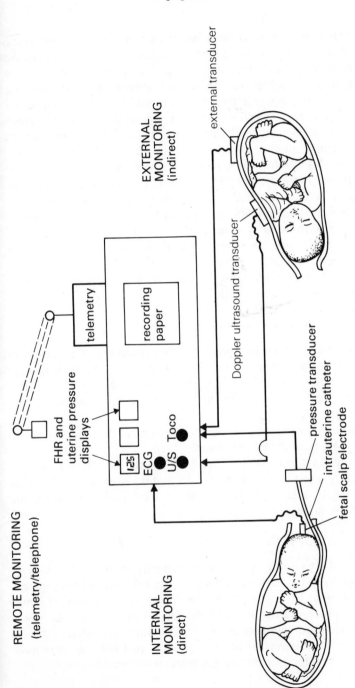

Fig. 2.1 Methods of monitoring FHR and uterine activity

of FHR monitors an attempt has been made to overcome these disadvantages by employing microprocessors and autoregulation — the process used to identify and analyse signals buried in noise — in order to achieve an FHR trace almost identical with that obtained from a direct fetal ECG. In addition, new wide-beam ultrasound transducers require less repositioning and therefore give less discomfort to the mother in labour. These innovations may mean less use of invasive fetal scalp electrodes in the future. Nevertheless, older FHR monitors are in use in many labour wards and therefore the limitations of external ultrasound compared with direct fetal ECG monitoring should be remembered.

It has not been possible to monitor twins adequately using two separate ultrasound systems as they interfere with one another. Fortunately some monitors have dual heart rate monitoring whereby an ultrasound trace and a direct ECG trace can be obtained simultaneously on the same machine, making the monitoring of twins in labour easier.

Fetal ultrasound telemetry

Some monitors have the facility to allow continuous fetal monitoring without confining the patient to bed, thus permitting her the freedom to walk around in early labour if she so wishes. The patient carries a small, pocket-sized telemetry transmitter. Information regarding both fetal heart and uterine activity can be transmitted to a remote telemetry receiver and then processed by a fetal monitor in the usual fashion.

Telephonic transmission of fetal heart and uterine activity signals to a receiver in the maternity unit is also now possible, thus allowing a degree of monitoring of fetal well-being from the patient's home.

Abdominal ECG

The fetal ECG may be obtained indirectly by the application of electrodes to the maternal abdomen. By this method both maternal and fetal ECG complexes are obtained. The maternal signal can be processed out to leave the fetal signal and should give a more accurate representation of FHR variability than external Doppler ultrasound. Although a number of FHR monitors have this facility it tends to be unreliable and is not used routinely.

DIRECT ELECTRONIC FHR MONITORING

This is the most widely used method for continuous FHR monitoring during labour and delivery. An electrode is attached to the fetal presenting part following rupture of the membranes. The electrode should be applied over a bony part of the fetal skull and not over suture lines or fontanelles, and should not be used with a face presentation. The electrode can normally be applied after the cervix has dilated to 1 to 2 cm. This method of monitoring gives the most accurate FHR recording as it detects and measures instantaneous (beat-to-beat) FHR. The FHR trace obtained is not a straight line but a 'jittery' one. This is because the interval between beats varies. The better the machine, the more accurate will be the assessment of the FHR variability, which is an important sign of fetal well-being.

Uterine Activity

Traditionally, the frequency and strength of uterine contractions have been assessed clinically by abdominal palpation. This method however requires the continuous presence of the midwife and can be inaccurate. A continuous record of uterine activity can be obtained either indirectly via an external transducer (tocodynamometer) attached to the maternal abdomen or directly via a catheter inserted transcervically into the uterine cavity (Fig. 2.1).

EXTERNAL (INDIRECT) UTERINE ACTIVITY MEASUREMENT

The transducer is generally attached over the fundus, which tightens with each contraction, causing pressure on the transducer, and the uterine activity is then displayed on the trace. This method is not ideal, however, as although information is obtained regarding the frequency and duration of contractions it is of little help in assessing the intensity of the contraction. In addition, the mother often finds the belt that encircles the abdomen uncomfortable. Changes in belt tension caused by maternal movement mean that frequent adjustments of transducer position are required.

INTERNAL (DIRECT) UTERINE ACTIVITY MEASUREMENT

Direct monitoring of uterine activity may be achieved using a disposable fluid-filled catheter connected to an external transducer or a catheter with a small transducer at its tip. The catheters are passed transcervically into the uterine cavity.

The system can be calibrated, allowing measurement of basal uterine tone as well as the absolute strength of contractions. It also gives a more reliable recording of uterine activity than external monitoring and more accurately indicates the start and finish of contractions, allowing better interpretation of periodic FHR changes. Although rather an invasive technique for routine monitoring in labour, it is helpful where accurate assessment of the strength of contractions is important, e.g. in patients with a previous caesarean section, especially where oxytocin is employed, and in very obese patients where external monitoring and abdominal palpation have been unhelpful. It is also useful in monitoring the growth-retarded fetus, which is more prone to distress in labour, and where oxytocin is used in a grand multiparous patient.

This technique can only be used following rupture of the membranes and care must be taken with the insertion of the cannula, as perforation of the uterus and placental vessels has been reported.

Chart Paper

Figure 2.2 shows a typical example of chart paper currently in use. One page length of the chart is 10 centimetres.

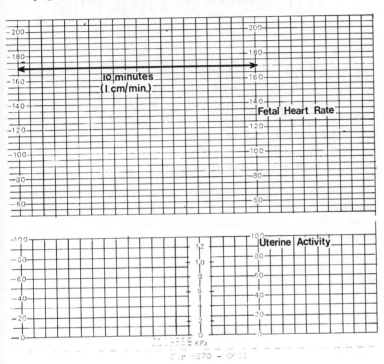

Fig. 2.2

The fetal heart rate is recorded on the upper portion of the paper and the scale is 50–210 divisions.

Uterine activity is recorded on the lower portion and this can be calibrated to give an accurate assessment of intrauterine pressure when an intrauterine pressure transducer is employed.

The normal chart speed employed in the UK is 1 centimetre per minute.

3

Terminology and Reporting

The interpretation of FHR traces and the ability to communicate this assessment of fetal well-being to others is one of the most difficult problems facing the newly appointed houseman in obstetrics. It is important therefore that a standard terminology and method of reporting is used.

Intrapartum FHR Monitoring

The terminology discussed below is based on the classification published by the American College of Obstetricians and Gynecologists in 1975 (*Technical Bulletin* No. 32), and is gaining increasing acceptance.

BASELINE FHR

The baseline FHR is the rate (in beats per minute — b.p.m.) at which the heart is set for most of a 10-minute period.

Normal		120–160 b.p.m.
Tachycardia	mild	161–180 b.p.m.
	severe	>180 b.p.m.
Bradycardia	mild	100–119 b.p.m.
	severe	<100 b.p.m.

Baseline tachycardia

A fetal tachycardia can result from a variety of causes:

1. In some cases of fetal asphyxia. However, where asphyxia is present the baseline tachycardia will be complicated by a reduction or absence of variability and/or the presence of decelerations.

   An uncomplicated baseline tachycardia with good variability would not be considered a sinister pattern.

A fetal tachycardia is occasionally seen on recovery from asphyxial stress, e.g. a large deceleration in the FHR is sometimes followed by a baseline tachycardia and is probably due to the release of catecholamines from the sympathetic nervous system and the adrenal medulla when the fetus is subjected to stress.
2. Maternal or fetal infection, e.g. chorioamnionitis.
3. Drug treatment, e.g. β-adrenergic agents used in an attempt to arrest preterm labour.
4. Extreme prematurity, when the parasympathetic nervous system is not so well developed.
5. Fetal tachyarrhythmias.
6. Thyrotoxicosis.

Baseline bradycardia

A mild bradycardia with good variability may be benign and not an indication of hypoxia. Alternatively, it may represent mild hypoxia that is being well compensated for by the fetus.

A severe bradycardia is a more serious prognostic sign and indicates that the fetus is failing to compensate (it is recognised by diminishing and eventually absent FHR variability). A bradycardia of < 80 b.p.m. will almost certainly result in fetal asphyxia unless action is taken.

Fetal bradycardia can also be due to cardiac conduction defects, e.g. heart block.

BASELINE FHR VARIABILITY

Variability can be described as short- or long-term.

Short-term variability (STV)

This is due to the varying beat-to-beat change (the R–R interval of the fetal ECG) in the fetal heart. It is obtained by direct FHR monitoring via a fetal scalp electrode, although the latest machines can give a close approximation to STV via an external ultrasound transducer. However, many machines in use at present are unable to give a true STV when Doppler ultrasound monitoring is used.

Long-term variability (LTV)

This represents changes in the baseline rate that have a frequency of 2–6 cycles per minute and amplitude of 6–10 b.p.m.

In practice, as both types of variability occur together, when assessing an FHR trace a distinction between STV and LTV is not normally made. The trace is described as merely having normal, reduced or absent variability. As mentioned in Chapter 2, external ultrasound monitoring may give a false impression of variability because of interference from movements other than fetal heart rate motion.

The presence of variability indicates an intact fetal nervous system and as outlined in Fig. 1.1 is the product of many different influences. Normal FHR variability is a very important sign of fetal well-being.

FHR variability may be diminished or absent in the presence of cerebral or myocardial asphyxia. Non-asphyxial causes of reduced variability are:

— Drugs, e.g. pethidine, morphine, diazepam.
— The rest phase of fetal rest–activity cycles.
— Rarely, defects in fetal cardiac conduction, e.g. heart block.

PERIODIC CHANGES IN FHR

These are defined as changes in the FHR that occur in relationship to uterine contractions.

Accelerations

These are transient increases in the FHR lasting less than 10 minutes. Their presence is a good prognostic sign.

Decelerations (Fig. 3.1)

Decelerations cause the most confusion in definition and interpretation. This is mainly the result of the development of two separate classifications.

Caldeyro-Barcia identified Type I and Type II decelerations, whereas Hon classified decelerations into early, variable and late. It is often considered that Type I decelerations are benign and only Type II serious. However, some decelerations labelled as Type I are in fact variable decelerations, very likely due to cord compression, which if allowed to continue could result in fetal asphyxia.

A comparison of the two classifications is shown in Table 3.1.

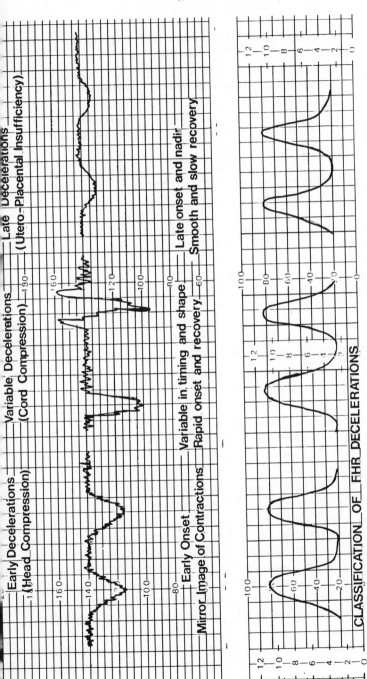

Fig. 3.1   Classification of FHR decelerations

Table 3.1   A comparison of the Hon and Caldeyro-Barcia classifications
of FHR decelerations

Hon classification	Clinical association	Caldeyro-Barcia classification
Early deceleration	Head compression	Type I dip
Late deceleration	Uteroplacental insufficiency	Type II dip
Variable deceleration	Cord compression	Various combinations of Type I and Type II

Early decelerations — head compression

These reflect the shape of uterine contractions and are usually
repetitive. The onset, maximal fall and recovery are coincident
with the onset, peak and end of contraction. These decelerations
are considered benign and are thought to be due to head compression. They are not nearly as common as variable decelerations.

Variable decelerations — cord compression

These decelerations are variable in onset in relation to the
contractions, variable in amplitude and duration, and tend to be
non-repetitive. In contrast to early and late decelerations the
change in FHR is rapid in both onset and recovery.

Variable decelerations are thought to be due to a reflex response to the sudden rise in blood pressure as a result of umbilical
cord compression.

These decelerations are very common in labour and where they
are of short duration and rapid recovery and in the presence of
good variability they indicate a normal physiological response to
cord compression and are considered benign. A mild respiratory
acidosis probably develops which recovers rapidly with the release
of cord compression. However, when they become severe (i.e.
below 60 b.p.m., 60 b.p.m. below baseline FHR, or longer than 60
seconds' duration — 'Rule of Sixties') and frequent, a metabolic
acidosis will eventually develop and the fetus may become compromised.

During labour mild variable decelerations may become deeper,
more prolonged and show a slow recovery to the baseline. This
progression in the severity of variable decelerations can indicate a
deterioration in the fetal condition and under these circumstances
a fetal scalp pH would be indicated.

Late decelerations — utero-placental insufficiency

The decelerations are often smooth and the onset, nadir and recovery are late in relation to the onset, peak and completion of the contraction.

Persistent late decelerations, especially in the presence of reduced variability, are a poor prognostic sign. They are due to uteroplacental insufficiency and reflect inadequate cerebral and myocardial oxygenation.

Initially, late decelerations may be very shallow and detection therefore depends upon careful observation. As the fetal condition deteriorates the decelerations become deeper and variability disappears.

Combined patterns

Such patterns are difficult to define but contain mixtures of the above.

Interpretation of the patterns is often very difficult, even to experts in the field, and only after fetal scalp blood sampling can the fetal status be correctly assessed.

RARE FHR PATTERNS

Sinusoidal pattern

A regular, smooth sine wave with a frequency of 3 to 6 per minute and an amplitude range of 5–30 b.p.m.

The cause of this pattern is unknown but has been associated with rhesus isoimmunisation, fetal anaemia and asphyxia. If this sinusoidal pattern is prolonged, and especially if it is accompanied by a reduction in variability, then a fetal scalp sample should be performed.

Saltatory pattern — 'excessive' variability

This bizarre pattern is occasionally seen where the variability seems excessive (amplitude greater than 25 b.p.m.). The cause of this excessive variability and its significance are uncertain. There is some evidence to suggest it may be associated with mild fetal acidosis and if it is persistent then a fetal blood sample would seem indicated.

When worrying decelerations develop a search should be made to try and find a correctable cause and this is dealt with in Chapter 7.

Reporting of Intrapartum Traces

A consistent method of reporting is important and the following is recommended:

1. *Baseline heart rate*	Normal, tachycardia, brady-cardia.
2. *Variability*	Normal, reduced or absent.

3. *Periodic changes*	Accelerations
	Decelerations — early
	              — variable
	              — late
	              — mixed patterns.

4. *Uterine contractions*	The classification of periodic FHR changes is impossible without an accurate assessment of uterine activity.
5. *Clinical progress*	The rate of deterioration in the FHR trace should be assessed in association with progress in labour. An FBS will give an indication of fetal pH and base deficit and will help in deciding whether to allow labour to continue. ünue.

NB: Careful notation of the FHR is essential and will facilitate interpretation. The patient's blood pressure and position, the administration of drugs, and the times of and findings at vaginal examinations should be noted on the trace where appropriate.

Antepartum FHR Monitoring

The antenatal cardiotocograph (CTG) involves the external monitoring of FHR variability and the occurrence of accelerations in response to fetal movement and/or uterine activity. The presence of accelerations in association with fetal movements is considered an important sign of fetal well-being.

Antepartum FHR traces are most commonly obtained using an ultrasound transducer. Although tests have been developed that stress the fetus (e.g. the contraction stress test or CST, whereby oxytocin is administered to the mother to provoke uterine contractions in order to assess the fetal response), it is the non-stress test (NST) that is by far the most commonly employed.

At present the NST is the only routinely available method of identifying the 'hypoxic' fetus in the antenatal period.

INDICATIONS FOR THE NST

There are many possible indications to perform an antenatal CTG, the most common being suspected growth retardation (IUGR), decreased fetal movements, post dates, maternal hypertension, maternal diabetes mellitus and bad obstetric history.

DURATION OF THE NST

Fetal rest cycles are of the order of 20 to 40 minutes' duration and therefore at least 20 minutes of good-quality tracing is required before a correct interpretation can be made.

INTERPRETATION OF THE NST

In the interpretation of antenatal CTGs the usual order of reporting can be employed, i.e. considering the baseline, the FHR variability and periodic changes.

The traces are generally classified as reactive or non-reactive, and the typical features are outlined in Table 3.2.

Table 3.2   Interpretation of the antenatal CTG

	Reactive	Non-reactive
Baseline	Normal range	May or may not be in normal range
Variability	Normal	Reduced or absent
Periodic changes	2 or more accelerations (greater than 15 b.p.m. and lasting 15 seconds) in response to fetal movement in a 10-minute test period*	No accelerations

*The number of accelerations required for a reactive trace varies from institution to institution.

A reactive trace is associated with a good fetal outcome, whereas a non-reactive trace may indicate a compromised fetus.

Where a 20-minute antenatal CTG is non-reactive or does not fulfil the criteria of a reactive trace, the period of observation should be extended for a further 20 minutes, as the initial test may have corresponded with a fetal rest cycle. Manual manipulation of the fetus may 'wake' the fetus up and thus give a reactive trace.

Where the CTG is persistently non-reactive, especially when there are no fetal movements, the case should be referred to a senior colleague for review. Unfortunately there is a high false-positive rate with the non-reactive CTG, and therefore careful consideration is required before contemplating intervention. If no immediate action is contemplated then the CTG will probably be repeated later that same day or the following morning.

NB: The *presence of decelerations* in an antenatal CTG is often a serious prognostic sign and again critical review at a senior level is required.

FREQUENCY OF THE NST

It is difficult to give exact guidelines here, as the frequency of the test will depend on the extent of concern for the well-being of a particular fetus. Twice-weekly CTGs are adequate for most cases, although daily or even more frequent testing may be required in a high-risk situation. Unfortunately, very occasionally a fetal death has occurred within 24 hours of a normal reactive CTG; therefore even daily CTG testing will not predict all fetal deaths.

It should be remembered that an antenatal CTG only gives information about a fetus at the time of the test and cannot predict a subsequent sudden event such as abruptio or a cord accident.

HOW EARLY SHOULD NST COMMENCE?

It would seem logical to start monitoring a fetus by CTGs when it has reached a gestational age at which intervention and delivery in the fetal interest would be considered. This in turn would depend on the neonatal services available. The high false-positive rates of non-reactive traces should be borne in mind here, as should the higher incidence of non-reactive traces in the very preterm fetus.

Examples of normal and abnormal antenatal CTGs will be given in Chapter 4.

4

Antenatal Cardiotocography

Methodology

A brief explanation of the procedure and the reasoning behind the test should be given to the patient. There should be little in the way of interruptions and if necessary the patient should empty her bladder first. She should be comfortable and reclining on a bed or examination couch at an angle of 30°. In an effort to ensure uniformity of testing and interpretation, a fixed testing schedule should be employed, a duration of 20 minutes usually sufficing.

The ultrasound transducer should be placed over the area where the fetal heart is most audible after abdominal palpation and auscultation with a Pinard stethoscope. A coupling medium should be smeared over the transducer in contact with the maternal skin. The transducer is held in place by a belt device and a second belt is also used for the tocography transducer, which is in effect a simple strain-gauge. This is placed over the fundus of the uterus and set so that the monitor records a slight positive tracing in the absence of a contraction.

The patient participates in the recording by marking down all fetal movements felt, either directly or by pushing an event marker on the machine. It is important to ensure that any loss of transducer contact during the recording is kept to a minimum, as it invalidates the CTG, wastes nursing and patient time and can cause unnecessary maternal anxiety.

NORMAL FEATURES

Baseline fetal heart rate — within 120–160 b.p.m.

Accelerations of the fetal heart rate in response to fetal movements and uterine contractions

Good baseline variability

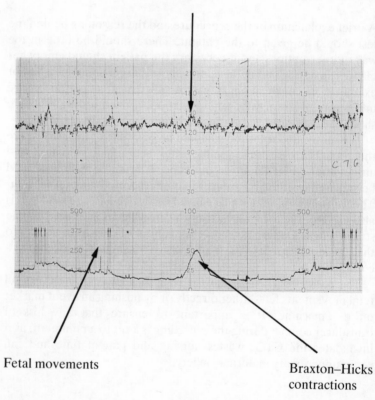

Fetal movements

Braxton–Hicks contractions

Fig. 4.1

It is important for the mother to record all fetal movements felt for the duration of the trace.

1. Baseline 130 b.p.m.
2. Variability normal.
3. Periodic changes — accelerations.
4. Uterine activity — Braxton–Hicks contractions.

The normal antenatal cardiotocograph: fetal rest cycle

Loss of baseline variability may be physiological and reflect a fetal 'sleep' cycle. These cycles tend to last less than 30 minutes and the dramatic change in the tracing below obtained in normal pregnancy demonstrates this well. Palpation of the abdomen can result in both an increase in variability and in accelerations of the fetal heart.

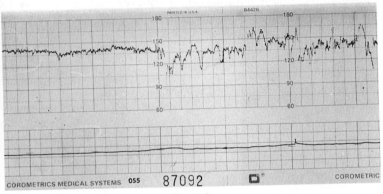

Fig. 4.2

It is important to determine the reason for a fetal heart rate recording that lacks variability. If the cause is a physiological rest cycle then a normal pattern should return after a further 20 minutes of monitoring. If this does not occur then the case should be reviewed at a more senior level.

> If an antenatal CTG shows no accelerations and/or poor variability over a 20-minute period then this should be continued for at least a further 20 minutes.

> A technically satisfactory CTG is
> essential before correct
> interpretation can be made.

A common source of artefact is electrical or signal error, which results in an unintelligible recording. This may arise from improper transducer placement or a faulty monitor. Such a recording provides no useful information whatsoever and serves only to generate anxiety in both patients and staff.

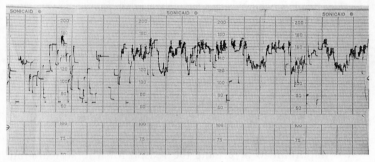

Fig. 4.3

1. Much loss of contact. Baseline indeterminate.
2. Variability indeterminate.
3. Periodic changes — unable to identify as accelerations or decelerations.
4. Neither uterine activity nor fetal movements recorded.

ABNORMAL FEATURES

Abnormal antenatal cardiotocography

Antenatal cardiotocography has a role in the monitoring of the high-risk fetus and will play a part in the decision to intervene.

Again it is important to differentiate between true decelerations of the fetal heart rate and loss of transducer contact. If any doubt exists then an attendant should sit with the patient to ensure an adequate and accurate recording.

> Any decelerations of the fetal heart, especially in the absence of variability in an antenatal CTG, are cause for concern.

Example (i)

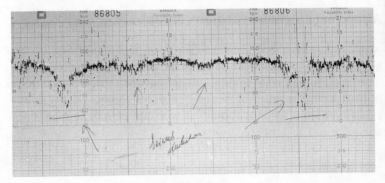

Fig. 4.4

1. Baseline, 150–160 b.p.m.
2. Variability reduced.
3. Decelerations.
4. No uterine activity.

Clinical details

Primigravida.
Clinically small-for-dates fetus.
Oligohydramnios.
Oestrogen–creatinine ratios beneath the tenth centile.
CTG at 30 weeks.
Emergency lower uterine segment caesarean section (LUSCS).
Birthweight 800 grams (g).
Umbilical artery (UA) pH 7.24.
Apgar scores 1[7], 5[9] (Time in minutes [Apgar score]).

Example (ii)

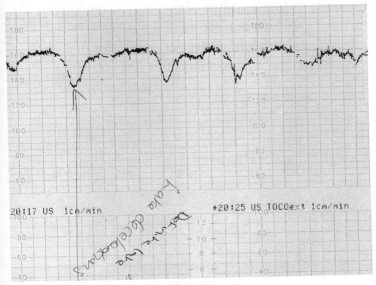

Fig. 4.5

1. Baseline 160 b.p.m.
2. Variability reduced.
3. Frequent decelerations.
4. No uterine activity recorded.

Clinical details

32 weeks' gestation.
Severe proteinuric hypertension; BP = 170/110 mmHg.
Symptomatic — headache, photophobia, vomiting.
Emergency LUSCS.
Birthweight 1.7 kg.
Poor condition at birth.
Apgar score 1[5].
UA pH = 6.9.

> Beware the shallow antenatal
> decelerations of the fetal heart,
> which may be missed but are as
> significant as deeper, more florid
> decelerations.

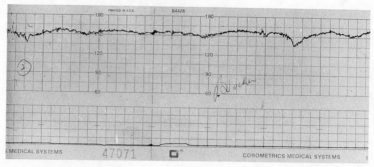

Fig. 4.6

1. Baseline 160 b.p.m.
2. Variability markedly reduced.
3. Shallow decelerations.
4. No uterine activity.

Clinical details

Multipara.
(Previous LUSCS at 33 weeks. Birthweight 1.82 kg. Neonatal death.)
Reduced fetal movements at 30 weeks.
CTGs show shallow decelerations and accompanying loss of variability.
Emergency LUSCS.
Male 1.05 kg.
Apgar 1[5].
Grossly infarcted placenta.
Baby alive and well following lengthy stay in neonatal unit.

A CTG should be part of the
assessment of a woman presenting
with abdominal pain or vaginal
bleeding in the third trimester of
pregnancy.

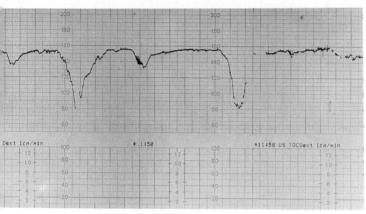

Fig. 4.7

1. Baseline 150 b.p.m.
2. Variability absent.
3. Decelerations.
4. Uterine activity not recorded.

Clinical details

Antenatal cardiotocography will help to establish fetal well-being in women presenting with abdominal pain. The above recording was seen at 31 weeks and represented a concealed abruption. The patient had had a previous caesarean section for a breech presentation. An emergency caesarean section was carried out on the basis of the above.

Umbilical artery pH 7.0.

Apgar 1[2].

Retroplacental clot.

Satisfactory neonatal outcome.

> A sudden reduction or cessation of
> fetal movements may be ominous
> and requires further assessment by
> antenatal cardiotocography.

The following two abnormal CTGs performed as a result of a diminution of fetal movements illustrate the importance of correct interpretation:

Example (i)

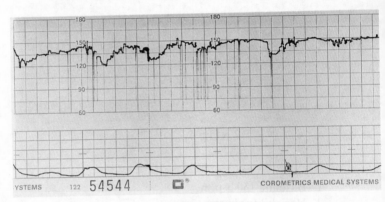

Fig. 4.8

1. Baseline 140–150 b.p.m.
2. Variability reduced.
3. Late decelerations.
4. Braxton–Hicks contractions.

Clinical details

19-year-old primigravida.
33 weeks. Pre-eclampsia.
Reduced fetal movements.
Decelerative CTG.
LUSCS.
Umbilical artery pH 7.18.
Baby alive and well following stay in neonatal unit.

Example (ii)

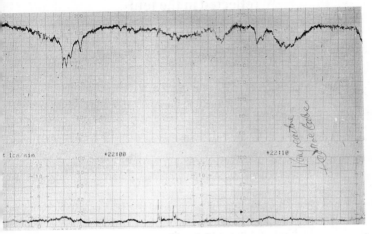

Fig. 4.9

1. Baseline 180–190 b.p.m.
2. Variability reduced.
3. Decelerations.
4. No uterine activity.

Clinical details

Primigravida at 39 weeks.
Admitted following a reduction in fetal movements.
CTG wrongly reported as very reactive.
Actually shows a fetal tachycardia with loss of variability and decelerations — a sinister pattern.
Note the absence of recorded fetal movements.
Readmitted 48 hours later with no fetal movements.
Intrauterine death.
Birthweight 1.98 kg.
Undiagnosed intrauterine growth retardation.

> If a CTG is not obviously normal
> always ask for another opinion at a
> more senior level.

Maternal ketoacidosis will be
reflected in the fetus.

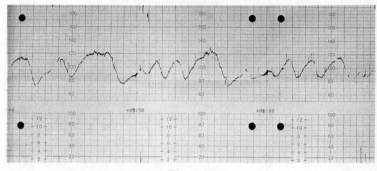

Fig. 4.10

1. No fixed baseline.
2. Variability absent.
3. Frequent prolonged decelerations.
4. No uterine activity.

Clinical details

Brittle diabetic admitted at 29 weeks with hyperglycaemia and ketosis.
Emergency LUSCS on basis of CTG.
Birthweight 1.5 kg.
Apgar 1[3].
Neonatal death.

Except in extreme prematurity, the same criteria for interpretation of CTGs should apply to both term and preterm fetuses, although accelerations tend to be less frequent and variability less in the latter. The preterm fetus can develop abnormal patterns more quickly and the severity of these progresses more rapidly.

Transient decelerations of short
duration due to umbilical cord
compression may be seen in the
presence of ruptured membranes.

In the presence of ruptured membranes, decelerations of short duration need not be ominous as long as they are of a transient nature and no other abnormal cardiotocographic features are present. *It is imperative* to establish no immediate fetal compromise and no deterioration in the fetal condition that would indicate the need to expedite delivery.

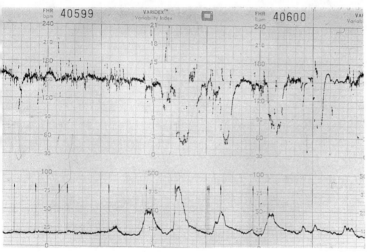

Fig. 4.11

INITIAL CTG

1. Baseline 150–160 b.p.m.
2. Variability difficult to interpret.
3. Decelerations.
4. Braxton–Hicks contractions.

Clinical details

Multigravida.
Preterm rupture of membranes.
Routine CTG at 28 weeks showing short decelerations of the fetal heart in response to Braxton–Hicks contractions.
Repeat CTGs were normal — Fig. 4.12.

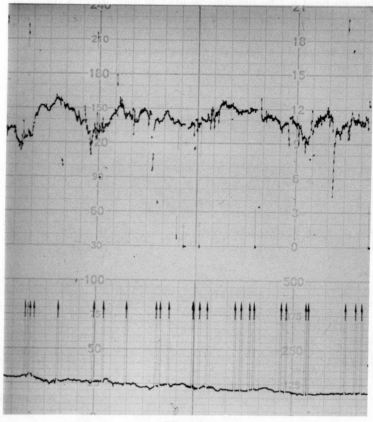

Fig. 4.12

REPEAT CTG

1. Baseline 120–130 b.p.m.
2. Variability normal.
3. Accelerations.
4. No contractions. Plentiful fetal movements.

Clinical details

The patient eventually laboured spontaneously in week 35 of her pregnancy with a good outcome. Birthweight 1.385 kg.

> Transient decelerations may be
> the first indicator of a
> deterioration in fetal condition.

The CTG changes associated with worsening fetal anoxia following transient decelerations are demonstrated by the following case:

Clinical details

Primigravida with recurrent antepartum haemorrhages and preterm rupture of membranes from 25 weeks.

(i) Antenatal CTG at 29 weeks showing a solitary deceleration in
    association with a Braxton–Hicks contraction.

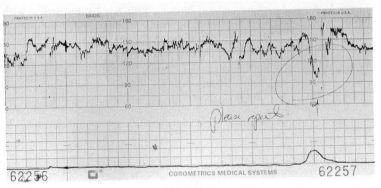

Fig. 4.13

1. Baseline 140–150 b.p.m.
2. Variability good.
3. Deceleration.
4. Solitary Braxton–Hicks contraction.

(ii) 17 hours later. Regular uterine contractions. Labour diagnosed. Prolonged deep deceleration.

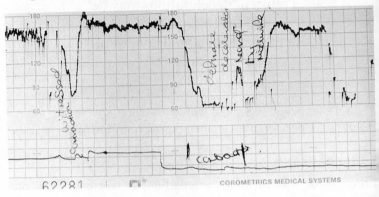

Fig. 4.14

1. Baseline 160 b.p.m.
2. Variability reduced.
3. Prolonged decelerations.
4. Contractions recorded manually.

(iii) CTG just prior to emergency LUSCS. Tachycardia with prolonged decelerations and absence of baseline variability. Female 950 g. Apgars 1^1, 5^3, 10^4. Perinatal death.

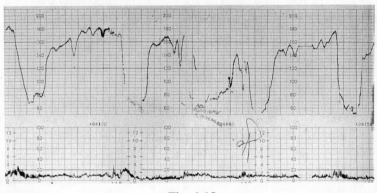

Fig. 4.15

1. Baseline 170–180 b.p.m.
2. Variability absent.
3. Deep prolonged decelerations.

> The stress of contractions may
> precipitate severe anoxia in a
> chronically anoxic fetus.

Cervical ripening and induction of labour can be achieved using prostaglandin E2. Prostaglandins instigate uterine contractions which may precipitate anoxia in a small-for-dates or preterm fetus who is less capable of coping with the resultant stress of contractions. This is reflected in an abnormal antenatal CTG.

Patients given prostaglandins for induction of labour or cervical ripening should have a CTG performed 30 minutes following administration for at least 20 minutes. Consideration should also be given to performing a CTG prior to cervical ripening. The need for this is illustrated by the following two CTGs.

Clinical details

Clinical small-for-dates primigravida at 37 weeks. Reduced fetal
movements.
Cervical os closed.
3 mg prostaglandin vaginal pessary inserted.

(i) CTG prior to prostaglandin administration

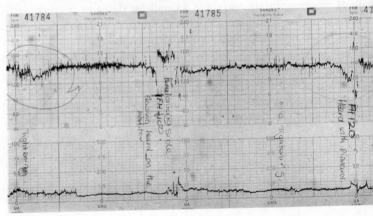

Fig. 4.16

1. Baseline 150 b.p.m.
2. Variability reduced.
3. Shallow decelerations.
4. Contractions recorded manually.

(ii) CTG after prostaglandin administration

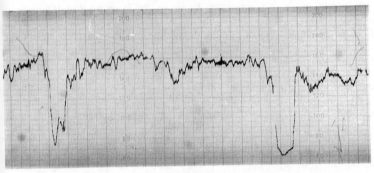

Fig. 4.17

1. Profound decelerations.
2. Emergency caesarean section.
3. Scanty liquor. Meconium present.
4. Birthweight 1.45 kg. UA pH 7.26. Apgars 1^5, 5^{10}.
5. Infarcted placenta.

Finally, it is important to remember that the cardiotocograph establishes the fetal condition only at the time of monitoring and it cannot predict any sudden insults that will affect fetal well-being.

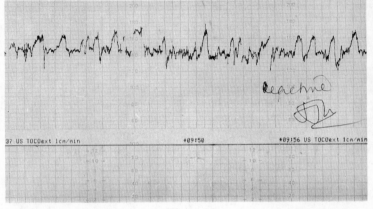

Fig. 4.18

1. Baseline 140 b.p.m.
2. Variability normal.
3. Accelerations.

Clinical details

Primigravida at 39 weeks.
Spontaneous rupture of membranes.
Clear liquor. Head engaged.
CTG excellent.
Transferred to labour ward the following day already established in labour.
Cervix 8 cm dilated.
Fetal heart not heard.
Fresh unexplained stillbirth. 3.14 kg.

5

Intrapartum Cardiotocography

FIRST STAGE OF LABOUR

A Normal CTG in Labour

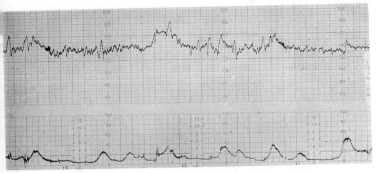

Fig. 5.1

1. Baseline 135 b.p.m.
2. Baseline variability normal.
3. Periodic changes: accelerations of the fetal heart in response to uterine contractions.
4. Uterine contractions as recorded by an external transducer.

Twins in labour

There are practical problems in the auscultation of twin fetuses in labour. The oncoming twin can be monitored electronically using a fetal scalp electrode, while the second twin, which has the higher perinatal mortality, is more difficult to monitor. Some electronic monitors will allow the superimposition of the second fetal heart rate using a Doppler ultrasound transducer onto the recording of the first twin. Such a system will highlight the two separate fetal heart rates, which is more difficult if two separate electronic monitors are used.

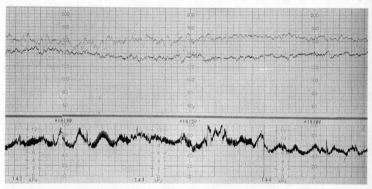

Fig. 5.2

TWIN I

1. Baseline 160–170 b.p.m.
2. Variability normal.
3. No decelerations.

TWIN II

1. Baseline 130–140 b.p.m.
2. Variability normal.
3. No decelerations.

Baseline changes

BRADYCARDIAS

> A *moderate* uncomplicated
> bradycardia with normal
> variability is not a sinister pattern.

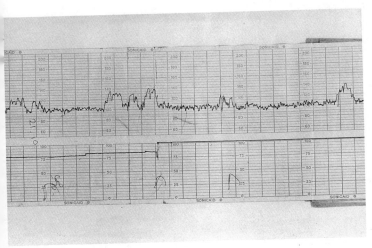

Fig. 5.3

1. Baseline 100 b.p.m.
2. Variability normal.
3. Accelerations.
4. Uterine activity not recorded adequately.

Idiopathic uncomplicated fetal bradycardia. No action required.
A fetal bradycardia that is complicated by decelerations or loss of
variability needs further assessment.

TACHYCARDIAS

> An uncomplicated fetal
> tachycardia is unlikely to be
> significant.

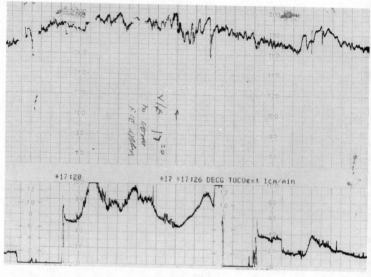

Fig. 5.4

1. Baseline 180–190 b.p.m.
2. Variability normal.
3. Accelerations.

Clinical details

Fetal tachycardia secondary to maternal pyrexia.
Uneventful outcome. Normal delivery. Apgar 1[9].
A fetal tachycardia of under 200 b.p.m. and uncomplicated by
other adverse cardiotocographic features is unlikely to be associated with fetal compromise. A rapid rate may decrease the
recordable variability to some extent.

> ## A complicated tachycardia warrants further action.

Fetal hypoxia manifest by a fetal tachycardia (180–190 b.p.m.) and late decelerations in a growth-retarded fetus.

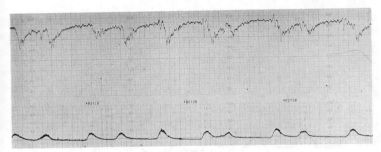

Fig. 5.5

1. Baseline 180–190 b.p.m.
2. Variability reduced.
3. Late decelerations.
4. Uterine contractions incoordinate.

Clinical details

Primigravida. Spontaneous labour at 38 weeks.
Meconium-stained liquor.
Emergency LUSCS.
Birthweight 2.32 kg.
Apgars 1^1, 5^3, 7^6.
5-week stay in neonatal unit.

A rise in baseline heart rate may
reflect a deterioration in the fetal
condition.

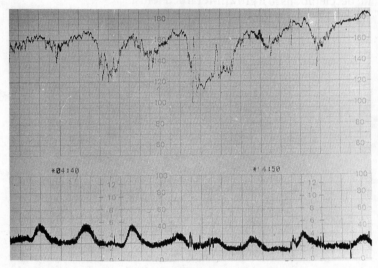

Fig. 5.6

1. Baseline progressively rising.
2. Variability decreasing.
3. Variable decelerations.
4. Contractions every 3 minutes.

Clinical details

Primigravida. Spontaneous labour at term.
CTG recording at 8 cm.
Fetal blood sampling pH 7.21, 7.18.
Emergency LUSCS.
Meconium noted.
Birthweight 3.39 kg.
Apgars 1[5], 5[9].
Umbilical artery pH 7.15.

Variability changes

REST–ACTIVITY CYCLES

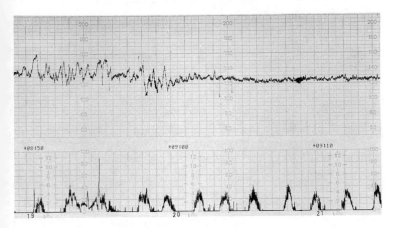

Fig. 5.7

Fetal rest cycles seen in the antenatal period also occur in labour.

DRUGS

> During labour decreased
> variability may result from drug
> administration, including opiates,
> anaesthetics or sedatives.

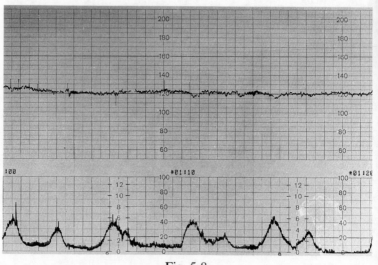

Fig. 5.8

1. Baseline 120 b.p.m.
2. Variability reduced.
3. No periodic changes.
4. Contractions every 2–3 minutes.

Reduced baseline variability following administration of pethidine in labour.

FETAL ASPHYXIA

> Absence of variability is a serious
> prognostic sign.

Marked loss of baseline variability associated with fetal asphyxia.

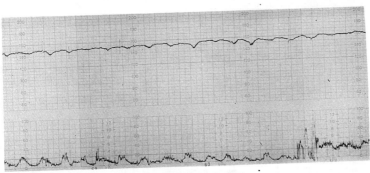

Fig. 5.9

1. Baseline rising progressively.
2. Variability absent.
3. Shallow late decelerations.
4. Frequent contractions.

Clinical details

Primigravida. Spontaneous labour at 38 weeks.
Fetal heart recording following artificial rupture of membranes
(ARM) at 2 cm dilatation.
Emergency LUSCS.
Birthweight 2.95 kg.
Apgars 1^5, 5^7, 10^8.
Retroplacental clot.
Anoxic brain damage.
Neonatal death.

Periodic changes

EARLY DECELERATIONS

> Early decelerations are a *mirror image* of the uterine activity pattern and alone are not sinister.

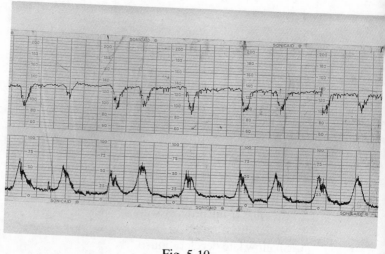

Fig. 5.10

1. Baseline 135 b.p.m.
2. Variability reduced.
3. Early decelerations.
4. Contractions every 3–4 minutes.

Clinical details

Variability improved within 30 minutes.
Normal delivery at term. Apgar 1[9].
Correct interpretation involving timing of decelerations in relation to contractions is vital.

VARIABLE DECELERATIONS

Example (i)

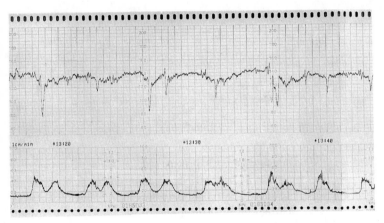

Fig. 5.11

1. Baseline 130–140 b.p.m.
2. Variability normal.
3. Mild variable decelerations.
4. Note the incoordinate uterine activity evidenced by coupling of the uterine contractions.

This would not be considered a sinister trace.

Clinical details

Normal delivery. Apgar 1[9]. Cord around neck.

Example (ii)

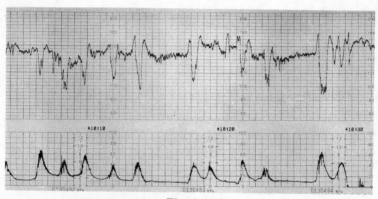

Fig. 5.12

1. Baseline 140–150 b.p.m.
2. Variability normal.
3. Frequent, variable decelerations that are short-lasting and return rapidly to the baseline. Shouldering present.

Clinical details

Spontaneous labour at term.
Normal delivery.
Birthweight 3.53 kg.
Apgars 1[6], 5[10].

Small accelerations often occur before or after variable decelerations; this is known as *shouldering*. In the presence of good variability this is considered benign. However, where the acceleration only follows the variable deceleration, i.e. overshoots the baseline with decreased or absent variability, this is often associated with fetal asphyxia.

Example (iii)

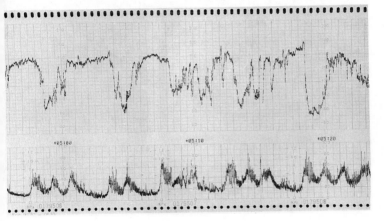

Fig. 5.13

1. Baseline 150 b.p.m.
2. Variability normal.
3. Frequent variable decelerations that are now more
   pronounced than in examples (i) and (ii). They are
   more prolonged and take longer to return to the
   baseline, and as such are more worrying.

Clinical details

A fetal scalp pH was performed and was normal (7.31).
A normal spontaneous delivery occurred with cord pH also =
7.31.
(The presence of good variability in this trace is reassuring.)

Example (iv)

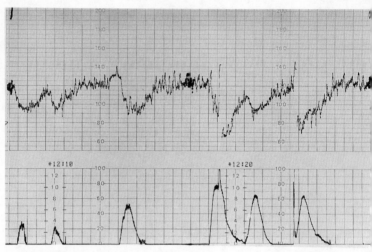

Fig. 5.14

1. Baseline 120 b.p.m.
2. Variability normal.
3. Deep variable decelerations with slow recovery to baseline.
4. Contractions incoordinate.

This slow recovery to the baseline is one step in the gradual deterioration of variable decelerations, although in this case the presence of good variability is reassuring.

Clinical details

Primigravida at 41 weeks' gestation.
Spontaneous rupture of membranes with meconium-stained liquor.
In view of slow recovery of variable decelerations, a caesarean section was performed at 2 cm dilatation.
Umbilical cord was round baby's neck but baby was in good condition at birth. Apgars 1[9], 5[10].

LATE DECELERATIONS

> Late decelerations are a serious
> prognostic sign.

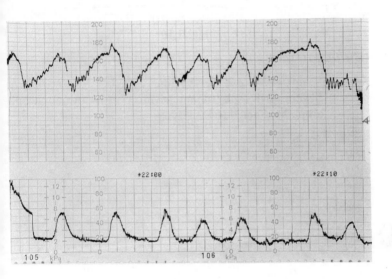

Fig. 5.15

1. Baseline 170 b.p.m.
2. Variability reduced.
3. Late decelerations.
4. Contractions every 3 minutes.

Clinical details

A fetal scalp sample was performed. pH = 7.12.
Emergency LUSCS at 7 cm dilatation.
Baby was in poor condition at birth and was intubated.
Apgars 1^2, 2^6, 5^8.

COMPLICATED PATTERNS

Asphyxia and perinatal deaths in a twin pregnancy.
Spontaneous labour at 35 weeks. Emergency LUSCS.

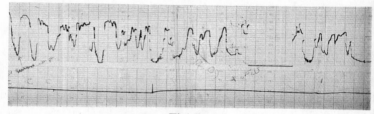

Fig. 5.16

Clinical details

Twin I   Scalp pH 7.0. 2.12 kg. Apgars 1^3, 3^6, 5^7.
Severe birth asphyxia and severe post-asphyxial encephalopathy. Died day 4.

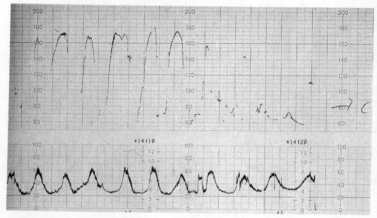

Fig. 5.17

Clinical details

Twin II   2.2 kg. Apgars 1^1, 3^1, 5^1.
Severe encephalopathy. Died day 3.

Both CTGs show changes associated with severe hypoxia.
    1. Baseline indeterminate.
    2. Variability absent.
    3. Severe decelerations.
    4. Contractions every 2 minutes.

Important clinical considerations

DECELERATIONS IN EARLY LABOUR

> A CTG in early labour may be
> crucial to the eventual outcome of
> the fetus.

Primigravida.
Regular contractions at 42 weeks.
No show. Intact membranes. Cervix 2 cm dilated.
CTG on admission shows pronounced decelerations.

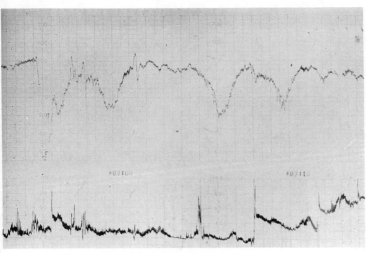

Fig. 5.18

1. Baseline 150 b.p.m.
2. Variability reduced.
3. Prolonged variable decelerations.
4. Uterine activity not recorded adequately.

Clinical details

ARM performed on basis of above. Scalp electrode applied.
Thick meconium drained.
Persistent decelerations and subsequent bradycardia.
Emergency LUSCS.
Birthweight 3.77 kg.
UA pH 7.11.
Apgars 1^3, 5^7, 10^9.

MECONIUM

The presence of meconium in the liquor may indicate fetal compromise.

> When the passage of meconium is confirmed following rupture of the membranes, electronic fetal heart monitoring should be employed.

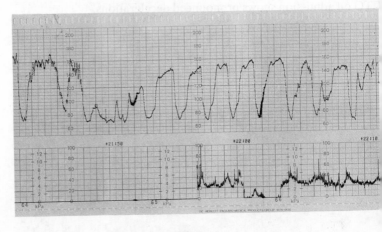

Fig. 5.19

1. Baseline 150–160 b.p.m.
2. Variability reduced with time.
3. Frequent deep decelerations.
4. Inadequate uterine monitoring.

Clinical details

Induction of labour at 42 weeks.
Thick meconium noted in labour.
Fetal blood sampling pH 6.90.
Emergency LUSCS.
Birthweight 2.65 kg.
Umbilical artery pH 7.08.

Cardiotocography should also be employed when the volume of liquor is either reduced or absent.

MATERNAL HYPOTENSION

Maternal hypotension will result in a reduction in uterine blood flow. This may lead to a hypoxic episode reflected by a fetal bradycardia. The insult may be transient if the cause of the hypotension is corrected. Once this is effected and normal oxygenation of the fetus resumed, one can expect the CTG to revert to the pattern prior to the insult.

Hypotension may result from sympathetic block, supine hypotension or hypovolaemic shock. In labour such episodes may be seen following an epidural top-up or other regional anaesthesia, a change in maternal position, use of a bedpan or vomiting.

> It is important to record relevant events on the CTG to aid overall assessment.

The following two examples illustrate the transient changes in patterns that can be seen following a fall in maternal blood pressure.

Example (i)

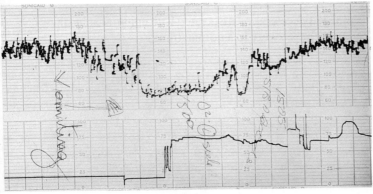

Fig. 5.20

Prolonged decelerations associated with a change in maternal position.

> The patient should not be nursed in the supine position in labour.

> # Women given an epidural anaesthetic in labour should be continuously monitored.

Example (ii)

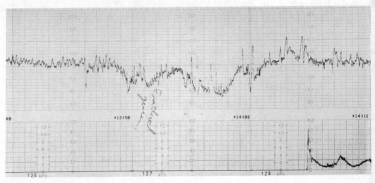

Fig. 5.21

Prolonged deceleration associated with epidural anaesthesia. Subsequent recovery to a normal trace.

UTERINE ACTIVITY

Uterine hypertonus will result in a fall in uterine blood flow and placental perfusion. Care must be taken in those labours where augmentation or induction is carried out using an intravenous oxytocin infusion when dosage requires to be titrated against response. The dose of oxytocin required once labour is in the accelerative phase is less than in the latent phase.

> Do not rely on the external transducer for information on the quality of uterine contractions.

In the absence of a functioning intrauterine catheter, contractions *must be palpated* for strength, duration and frequency, as well as resting uterine tone.

> Care must be taken to avoid
> uterine overstimulation in labour.

Example (i)

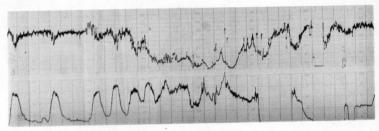

Fig. 5.22

Fetal bradycardia associated with oxytocin overstimulation. Recovery effected after discontinuing the oxytocin infusion.
Note the uterine activity pattern.

Example (ii)

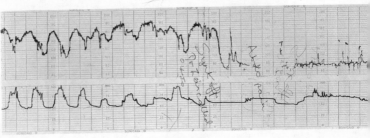

Fig. 5.23

Failure to recognise overstimulation or obstructed labour may result in severe bradycardia associated with uterine rupture. The above rupture at full dilatation resulted in a stillbirth. The patient had had three previous normal deliveries. She had an oxytocin infusion commenced after failing to progress at 5 cm dilatation. Full dilatation was achieved after 4 hours. Birthweight 3.46 kg. Note the late decelerations prior to the severe bradycardia at time of uterine rupture.

SECOND STAGE OF LABOUR

It is important to recognise that the fetus is subjected to different stresses in the second stage of labour. Although defined as the time between full dilatation and delivery of the fetus, the second stage can be divided into passive and active phases, depending on whether maternal pushing has started or not. This is especially evident if epidural anaesthesia is employed.

During the second stage there is a change in the uterine contraction pattern and an increase in compression of the fetal head. Uterine contractions become stronger and uterine pressure is further increased by the maternal efforts involved in bearing down. This does eventually lead to some impairment of fetal oxygenation and metabolic acidosis during the pushing phase, which may be well tolerated by the fetus.

The fetal heart responds to these changes so that a change in pattern may herald the onset of the second stage. Decelerations are commonly seen with contractions and alone do not necessarily mean hypoxia. Under these circumstances it is important to establish the presence of normal variability and baseline heart rate. A change in either is likely to indicate hypoxia and the need to intervene. The patterns may be difficult to interpret and lead to early delivery. Operative delivery is not without its risks to mother or fetus. Under these circumstances, and faced with the prospect of an early difficult delivery, a prompt senior opinion should be sought where possible.

The CTG below illustrates typical changes seen during the active pushing phase of the second stage of labour. Decelerations are noted with contractions with a normal baseline and good variability. The multi-spike artefact with the uterine contractions indicates maternal expulsive efforts as interpreted by the abdominal transducer and is a clue to when pushing has taken place.

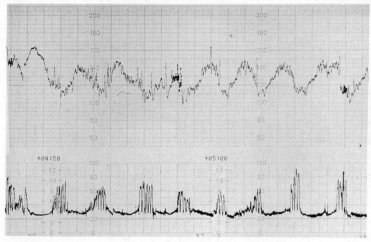

Fig. 5.24

1. Baseline 140–150 b.p.m.
2. Variability normal.
3. Decelerations with contractions.
4. Evidence of maternal effort with contractions.

Clinical details

Normal delivery.
Birthweight 3.02 kg.
Apgars 1^7, 5^9.

An ominous heart rate pattern may become evident only in the second stage of labour. The option of a fetal scalp pH should not be discarded because the patient has reached full dilatation.

The case below illustrates fetal heart changes as a result of fetal hypoxia in the second stage prior to commencement of pushing. Under these circumstances the CTG should be interpreted as in the first stage of labour.

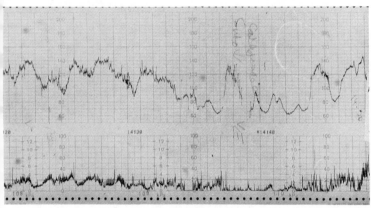

Fig. 5.25

1. Baseline 130–140 b.p.m.
2. Variability seen to be abolished with time.
3. Prolonged severe variable decelerations.
4. Uterine activity not adequately recorded.

Clinical details

Gestational diabetic. SROM at 36 weeks. Labour augmented with oxytocin infusion. Epidural anaesthesia. CTG at full dilatation.
Station + 3 cm.
Direct occipito-anterior position.
Easy forceps delivery.
Birthweight 2.35 kg. Cord pH 7.18. Apgars 1^2, 5^6, 10^9.

> In the presence of severe fetal
> distress, abdominal delivery may
> be safer than a potentially difficult
> operative vaginal delivery.

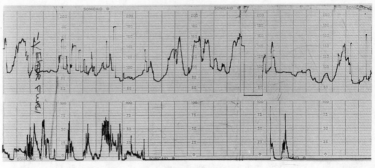

Fig. 5.26

1. Previous baseline 150–160 b.p.m. with change to
   complicated bradycardia 80–90 b.p.m.
2. Variability absent.
3. Complex decelerative pattern.

Clinical details

Primigravida.
Spontaneous labour at 38 weeks.
Full dilatation.
Right occipito-lateral. Caput + +. Moulding + +. Station 0.
Meconium + +.
Emergency caesarean section.
Birthweight 2.56 kg.
Apgars 1^2, 5^{10}.
UA pH 7.0.

> A severe fetal bradycardia in the
> second stage requires delivery.

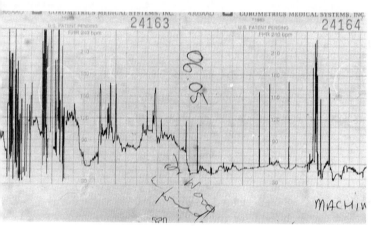

Fig. 5.27

1. Baseline 50–60 b.p.m.
2. Variability reduced.
3. Decelerations prior to bradycardia.

Clinical details

Spontaneous labour at 41 weeks.
Severe bradycardia and fresh meconium at full dilatation.
Mid-cavity forceps delivery.
Birthweight 3.01 kg.
Apgars 1^7, 5^9.

Intrapartum asphyxia in second stage leading to perinatal death:

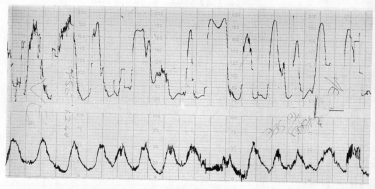

Fig. 5.28

1. No fixed baseline.
2. Variability absent.
3. Severe deep decelerations.
4. Uterine contractions every 2 minutes.

Clinical details

Primigravida aged 21.
Spontaneous labour at 38 weeks.
CTG at full dilatation shows a tachycardia with deep late decelerations and absence of variability.
Station + 2 cm.
Right occipito-posterior position.
Kiellands forceps delivery.
Meconium passed.
Cord tightly round neck.
Apgars 1^0, 5^1.
Perinatal death after 48 hours.

6

Diagnostic Pitfalls

Faulty signal

An inaccurate recording of the fetal heart rate as a result of a faulty signal pick-up may mask a significant fetal heart rate pattern. The following two CTGs were recorded sequentially in the same woman in labour, the first using Doppler, the second following application of a fetal scalp electrode. Note the clue in the first CTG, which is the entry recording the fetal heart rate as 170 b.p.m. on auscultation, as opposed to the apparent rate of 145 b.p.m. The recognition of an unsatisfactory Doppler recording in labour warrants application of a scalp electrode.

DOPPLER RECORDING

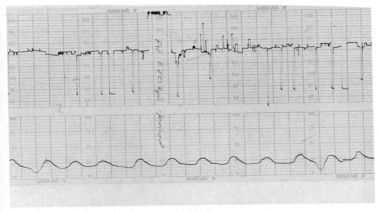

Fig. 6.1

The true recording pattern emerges on changing the monitoring technique to reveal a complicated tachycardia that warrants fetal blood sampling.

FSE RECORDING

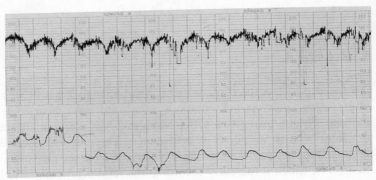

Fig. 6.2

1. True baseline 170 b.p.m.
2. Variability indeterminate
3. Late decelerations.
4. Uterine contractions every 2–3 minutes.

Scalp pH was 7.33.
Subsequent elective forceps for dural tap.
Apgar 1[9].

Baseline variability

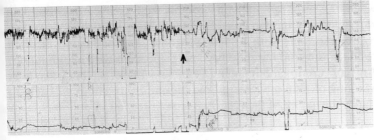

Fig. 6.3

Artificial 'jitter' on a Doppler ultrasound recording may be incorrectly interpreted as good baseline variability. The CTG above dramatically illustrates this point, showing a change in pattern on application of a fetal scalp electrode (arrowed).

Baseline heart rate

It may be difficult to identify the true baseline fetal heart rate and decide whether a normal rate is exhibiting marked accelerations or whether this is an ominous complicated tachycardia. Baseline variability is helpful in this assessment as good variability is known to be associated with a good prognosis and patience will often result in the true baseline becoming apparent within 20 minutes. Any concern in labour should be offset with fetal blood sampling. Marking of fetal movements and uterine contractions will help to clarify the nature of the CTG.

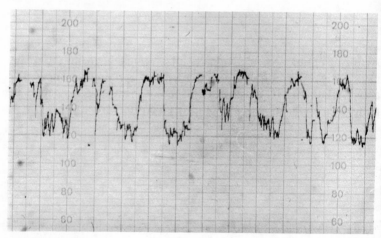

Fig. 6.4

The baseline here was correctly identified as being 130 b.p.m. within 15 minutes of the above pattern.

Twin pregnancies

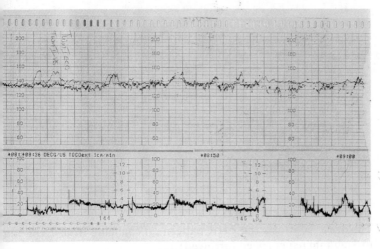

Fig. 6.5

A striking example of how twin fetal heart rates may be so similar that were the rates not superimposed and two individual monitors used, the attendant could be forgiven for thinking that only one fetus was being adequately monitored.

Paper speed

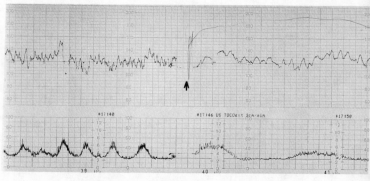

Fig. 6.6

This trace contrasts the FHR pattern on changing from 1 cm/min to 3 cm/min paper speed (arrowed).

A paper speed more rapid than 1 cm/min may result in apparent reduced variability and prolonged decelerations. The standard speed used in the United Kingdom is 1 cm/min.

Cardiac arrhythmias

> Fetal cardiac arrhythmias may
> result in highly abnormal fetal
> heart rate patterns.

Example (i)

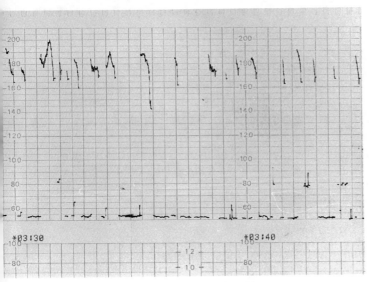

Fig. 6.7

Clinical details

38 weeks. Antenatal CTG.
Irregular fetal heart rate alternating between 150–200 b.p.m. and
50–60 b.p.m. No abnormality on cardiac ultrasound.
Emergency LUSCS.
Birthweight 2.82 kg.
Apgars 1^8, 5^9.
UA pH 7.26.
Irregular heart rate for the first 24 hours after delivery. Subse-
quently settled spontaneously to a normal rhythm.
No drug therapy required.

Example (ii)

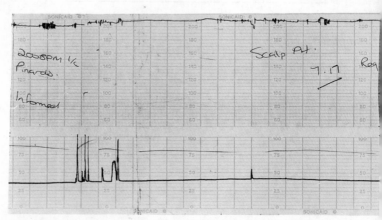

Fig. 6.8

Clinical details

Multigravida 42 weeks. Induction of labour.
Tachycardia $\geq$ 200 b.p.m.
Scalp pH 7.17 at full dilatation.
Midcavity forceps delivery.
Birthweight 4.88 kg.
Atrial flutter 2.1 block. Baby digitalised.

Fetal heart rates in tachyarrhythmias may exceed the upper limit of recording capability. Under these circumstances the machine may record a rate that is half that of the true rate. This halving artefact is seen only rarely but when it occurs the fetal heart rate may appear to be within normal limits.*

---

* A similar effect may be seen when the fetal heart rate is very slow and the recorded rate is seen to double (*doubling*).

Maternal signal transmission

A maternal signal can be transmitted by Doppler in the course of antenatal or intrapartum monitoring. The difference in maternal and fetal heart rates can result in an incorrect interpretation of what would appear to be an apparent fetal bradycardia when the signal pick-up changes from fetal to maternal sources.

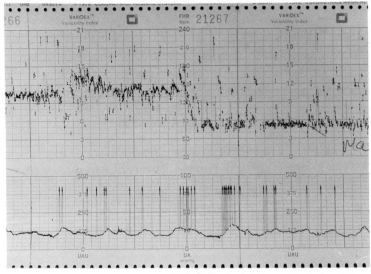

Fig. 6.9

Fetal heart rate: 130–140 b.p.m.
Maternal heart rate: 80 b.p.m.
Change in signal associated with burst of fetal activity.

In such cases the maternal pulse should be checked and the fetal heart auscultated to establish the true nature of the recording. A maternal tachycardia may impart a false sense of security as the rate would be compatible with the normal fetal heart rate and accelerations may be seen with contractions. Incorrect application of a fetal scalp electrode (e.g. to the cervix) will also record the maternal rate.

A maternal signal can be recorded as a result of transmission in cases of intrauterine death and the examples overleaf illustrate how this can occur using both Doppler and direct fetal monitoring.

Example (i) Doppler

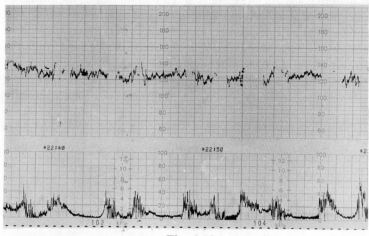

Fig. 6.10

CTG in labour (Doppler). Normal delivery of macerated stillbirth.

Example (ii) FSE

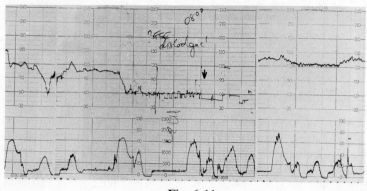

Fig. 6.11

(Courtesy A.Murray)

Transmission of maternal heart rate via a fetal scalp electrode following fetal death (arrowed). The maternal tachycardia was associated with a hydralazine infusion.

Unusual patterns

There are occasions when bizarre patterns are seen that do not readily fit into any of the categories previously described.

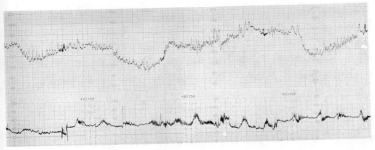

Fig. 6.12

The above patient laboured spontaneously at term and had meconium-stained liquor. The CTG shows a wandering baseline that could be interpreted as broad late decelerations. Note that the baseline variability is excellent. Fetal scalp pH is useful to clarify matters and in this case was 7.35. The CTG subsequently reverted to a more familiar normal pattern and a normal delivery of a healthy female resulted. Apgars $1^7, 7^9$.

7

Therapeutic Measures

Some of the abnormalities of the fetal heart rate previously described, while not being precise indicators of hypoxia, will be highly suggestive of fetal compromise. Abnormal patterns demand a search for a cause. These patterns can be subdivided into changes that are transient and those that are more persistent. The former arise as a result of a temporary insult to the fetus and can by their very nature be rectified, especially if the precipitating cause is identified. Nevertheless, even if the specific cause is not known, basic measures will often alleviate abnormalities of the fetal heart rate (Table 7.1). If a well-compensated fetus suffers an acute asphyxial insult there is every possibility of abolishing the abnormal heart rate pattern. Persistent and worsening abnormal changes are likely to be caused by more significant factors that will be less easily correctable and be more likely to require delivery of the fetus. Once placental reserve is surpassed so that decreases in uterine blood flow with contractions cannot be tolerated, it is unlikely that any measures will result in the abolition of the resultant decelerations. The measures described can however alleviate the clinical situation to some extent while preparations for delivery are under way.

Maternal posture in labour is important with regard both to supine hypotension and to compression of the umbilical cord or placental bed. The former is associated with prolonged decelerations, the latter with variable decelerations. Compression of the inferior vena cava by the gravid uterus will lead to a reduction in cardiac output and a fall in blood pressure. This results in a reduction in the uteroplacental circulation. Prevention is more important than correction under these circumstances and the patient should not lie in the supine position in labour. A wedge can be placed beneath the mattress to displace the uterus. The left lateral position is usually preferable, although the fetal heart may respond best when the patient is on her right side.

After rupture of the membranes the umbilical cord is liable to be subject to compression, thereby reducing fetal blood flow and oxygenation. The consequent variable decelerations may not be significant in the short term but efforts should be made to abolish them. Normally, mild to moderate variable decelerations can be well tolerated by the fetus for some time. However, if these are severe or associated with changes in baseline rate or variability then even the well-grown fetus with adequate placental function will be affected. Changing maternal posture under these circumstances is suggested in order to redistribute the mechanical forces causing compression of the umbilical cord.

A *vaginal examination* will help to exclude prolapse of the cord and may reveal surprisingly rapid progress in labour. The second stage may thereby be diagnosed, allowing the operator the option of a vaginal delivery if necessary.

Table 7.1 Action list for an abnormal CTG in labour

Aim to improve fetal oxygenation, relieve acidosis and abolish the abnormal fetal heart rate pattern.

1. Change maternal posture.
2. Check blood pressure. Correct hypotension.
3. Improve maternal oxygenation.
4. Assess uterine activity. Discontinue oxytocin infusion.
5. Vaginal examination. Exclude cord prolapse and assess progress in labour.
6. Consider fetal blood sampling or operative delivery.

Although supine hypotension has been referred to, hypotension from any cause will lead to a fall in the uteroplacental circulation. The accompanying fetal heart rate changes tend to be transient as long as the cause is corrected. By restoring the maternal arterial pressure, the intervillous space blood flow will be raised.

Epidural anaesthesia not only affects the autonomic nerve supply; the local anaesthetics used are also rapidly absorbed from the extradural space into the maternal circulation and thence to the fetal circulation via the placenta. The heart rate changes can vary from profound prolonged decelerations to loss of baseline variability and can be seen after an epidural top-up. This highlights the potential problems that can result from excessive or too rapid administration of the local anaesthetic. It is therefore important to maintain an intravenous infusion and also to monitor the fetus with care in the presence of an epidural anaesthetic.

Maternal blood pressure should always be checked after a top-up. The management of hypotension after a top-up should initially involve an alteration in maternal posture followed if necessary by the rapid intravenous infusion of 500 ml of full-strength Hartmann's solution or alternatively a colloidal or crystalloid preparation. In the absence of a response to these basic measures, resuscitation should be continued with the help of the resident anaesthetist by giving further fluids and ephedrine intravenously. Ephedrine can be given slowly in 3–5 mg aliquots until a response is obtained and may be subsequently given as an intramuscular dose or slow intravenous infusion.

In an attempt to improve fetal oxygenation in the presence of hypoxic CTG changes, *oxygen* should be administered to the mother either by mask or via a nasal cannula. This raises the materno-fetal pO_2 gradient and will potentially increase the maternofetal oxygen transfer where there is hypoxia.

Uterine activity has to be closely monitored in labour, as overstimulation with oxytocin will result in hypoxic CTG changes. Even in the presence of fetal compromise unrelated to uterine overstimulation, the continuing of an oxytocin infusion may compound matters and worsen the fetal condition. Under the circumstances it is wise to discontinue the oxytocin infusion until fetal well-being is established, either by fetal blood sampling or by a return to a normal fetal heart rate pattern. By reducing the uterine activity the intervillous space will be better perfused and the periods between the stress of contractions will be lengthened. Active pushing may be best discouraged in the short term until fetal condition is established or delivery expedited. If there is uterine hyperstimulation in the form of a sustained uterine contraction, or as an interim measure prior to delivery, then a bolus dose of a sympathomimetic (e.g. ritodrine, 2 mg intravenously) may be given. This will relax the uterus and improve uterine blood flow.

The measures described should be carried out in a practised and systematic manner while the reasons for these actions are explained always to the patient. Changes in the fetal heart rate pattern may herald fetal hypoxia and this can potentially be corrected if the above procedures are adhered to.

There are known to be associations between abnormal fetal cardiotocographic patterns and fetal condition but these are by no means absolute. Although it is very helpful on many occasions, the value of cardiotocography is limited by the looseness of these associations and the rather poor predictive value of an abnormal CTG trace. This important point should be remembered when judging FHR traces retrospectively.

Index